Rhythms of the Week

Rhythms of the Week

And other Explorations of Time

Wolfgang Held

Floris Books

Translated by Matthew Barton

Part One first published in German as *Der siebenfache
Flügelschag der Seele* in 2004
Part Two taken from *Vier Minuten Sternenzeit*, first
published in Germany in 2006.
Both published by Verlag Freies Geistesleben.
Published in English by Floris Books in 2011
© 2004 & 2006 Verlag Freies Geistesleben & Urachhaus GmbH, Stuttgart
English version © Floris Books 2011

British CIP Data available

ISBN 978-086315-792-9

Printed in Poland

Acknowledgments

In particular I would like to thank Hartwig Schiller, whose remarks caused me to attend more carefully to the qualities of the days of the week, and my father, Berthold Held, whose stylistic suggestions proved very helpful.

Contents

Foreword — 00

Part One: Living with the Rhythm of the Week — 00 11

The Soul's Sevenfold Wingbeat — 00 13
Sunday: When Does the Week Begin? — 00 21
Monday: Attending to the New — 00 29
Tuesday: A Special Day for Mistakes — 00 37
Wednesday: Interest in What's Around You — 00 45
Thursday: Acting with Insight and Overview — 00 53
Friday: The Importance of What Seems Secondary — 00 61
Saturday: How Does the Old Enter the World? — 00 69

Part Two: Living with the Rhythms of Time — 00 77

The Equilibrium of the Present — 00 79
How Long Is the Present? — 00 83
Speed and Heart Rhythm — 00 87
How Long Does a Moment Last? — 00 91
The New Day Begins in the Evening — 00 95
From Discoverer to Philosopher in the Cycle of the Year — 00 97
The Will's Small and Great Rhythm — 00 101

Foreword

We have conquered space. Every last bit of land has been measured and even the furthest corners of the globe have been mapped and can be reached by some means of transport. Today's voyages of discovery no longer take place in physical space but in the dimension that still often confounds us: time. In the 21st century this is the terra incognita, the unknown realm. Whether in the temporal configurations of our biography or the rhythmic effect of times of day and seasons of the year on our psyche and physical organism, we are finding increasingly that time does not flow in a uniform way but is, rather, a fabric woven of the most varying, changing qualities. It is high time, perhaps, that we tried to notice it more, to understand and incorporate it into our lives with greater awareness.

Few things have such a decisive affect on our positive personal development as our individual relationship with time. A hundred years ago, the Austrian poet Ödön von Horváth lamented that he rarely found time for anything. If this makes us smile today it is because we still relate to it, in fact more so than ever.

In the 20th century, time-management advisers were largely the preserve of commerce and business, but today, increasingly, we are all faced by the vital question of our relationship to time. In the eighties, Gunther Hildebrand, a pioneer of modern rhythm research, stated that 'Every person today is caught in a chronobiological time conflict.' Our modern lives are such that we are frequently at odds with our organic rhythms and therefore continually weaken our own vitality. Of course none of us can avoid the hectic pace of things today. The question is therefore not how to avoid this life-sapping way of living but rather how to cope better with the arrhythmia of modern life and ultimately organize it in a masterful and musical way.

Rhythm is always the best way of structuring our time. To develop new rhythms in our own lives, it is worth exploring and learning about the many existing rhythms and inner qualities at work in temporal processes. By this means we can gain a relationship to time and, instead of battling against it, make it into our tool and ally.

The voyage of exploration into the structure of the seven-day week described in Part One of this book aims, like any good guidebook, to facilitate your own discoveries, helping to get a purchase on this fleeting element so that it can serve you better in daily life.

Part Two offers some insights into other rhythms of life, to help acquaint you better with time and its possibilities. It encourages you to explore some previously unknown rhythms and use them creatively in your life.

Wolfgang Held

1 | Living with the Rhythm of the Week

The Soul's Sevenfold Wingbeat

What underlies the
seven-day week?

Water and soul are related

Comparisons are often made between the human psyche and the sea. The ocean is as broad and unfathomable as the human soul, but they have something else in common too — movement. While it seems as if water is always set in motion by an external cause such as the wind, a closer look can tell us that movement is intrinsic to the nature of water itself. A simple test can illustrate this: if you let a trickle of water run down a sloping sheet of glass, the water will of course follow the slope, heeding gravity, but at the same time will also seek its own, winding and continually changing path. Water has a tendency to pulsate and move: an inner vivacity which, over long periods, gives rise to those wonderfully curving river meanders that engrave themselves into the landscape — as long as water is not compelled to flow in straight, man-made channels. Even when still, water is usually in movement or expecting movement: a gentle breeze is enough, the flap of a fin, and immediately water responds with rhythmic waves. It does, though, need some kind of external stimulus to begin to stir.

The sovereign soul

The human soul is related to these qualities. Every sensory impression or external stimulus can set our soul in motion, evoking inner response in the form of feelings, thoughts or even actions. It is not for nothing that we say someone is 'cold' if they do not respond to outward occurrences with interest and involvement. They appear, then, to be like frozen water that likewise loses its 'love of movement,' its receptive sensitivity.

But whereas water is reliant on outer stimulus to begin pulsing and swirling, we are capable of initiating movement without external cause, entirely out of ourselves. At such times we can experience everything external as distraction, and become aware of hidden inner movement within us. This capacity is wonderfully depicted in the figure of Baron Munchhausen, who pulls himself up by his own tuft of hair to free himself from a swamp. The soul can find its own impetus for movement and development, and there is probably no religion in the world that does not acknowledge this capacity as the soul's sovereign or regal nature. Language itself contains much wisdom: we speak both of raising and deepening in relation to the ego's self-initiating power of impetus, whether through reflection, meditation or prayer. At such times the soul resembles a calm mountain lake, reflecting the heavens yet also allowing us to see into its depths.

The soul swings back and forth between two extremes — the stronger it does so the better — finding stimulus and renewal in the outer world then returning home to be entirely centred in itself. The more we are able to withdraw into our own thoughts with a good book, a thought-provoking saying or any other content of reflection — even for just a few minutes each day — the more interest and participation we can call upon when meeting others, engaging with new ideas or going out into nature.

Those who practise such things will notice that on some days of the week they succeed less well than on others. For instance, it seems harder to focus on oneself on Wednesdays, while on Thursdays it is easier to make decisions and meet challenges. Why is this?

The weekly rhythm

The week has a remarkable rhythm that does not precisely accord either with the month or the year: a particular date will always fall on different days. In purely commercial terms, the week is the least practical aspect of our temporal divisions into second, minute, hour, day, week, month and year. Yet most of humanity keeps faith with this sevenfold rhythm. Seen from the point of view of astronomy, the week is also an exception. Whereas the month is derived from the moon, and the day and the year from the sun's circuit, the week does not accord with any temporal division exemplified by the cosmos — except perhaps very roughly the four quarters of the moon at new moon, half moon and full moon.

What was it in ancient times that allowed the seven-day week, originating in Chaldea, to triumph over the many other ways that then existed of subdividing the month — such as the Sumerians' five-day week, the Romans' eight-day week, the Babylonians' nine-day week or the Egyptians' ten-day week? The answer lies in us human beings. Just as activity and passivity typically alternate during the course of a day, so that, for instance, we are generally least energetic between 1.30 and 2.30 p.m., the human soul likewise resonates from day to day in seven differing moods.

The astonishing thing is that these moods correspond to the qualities and character of the seven classical planets to which each day of the week was assigned in ancient Babylon around 4,000 years ago.

Investigating time today

To investigate time today in a way that takes its lead from the cosmos means both observing the typical character of a day of the week, and also examining the special qualities ascribed to the planet that supposedly governs it. This comparative view will help us understand why, for example, collaborating with others on Tuesday might be particularly challenging.

Knowing more about the qualities of each day of the week, and using these qualities so that we are most effective in what we do, can help us cope better with the demands of modern life and work. In the following chapters we will examine the typical characteristics of each day. This does not of course mean offering fixed prescriptions of any kind but rather giving stimulus to sharpen our perception of time's living, differentiated qualities. Thus each person can set about their own enquiries and reach their own conclusions. This may lead to discoveries such as that school tests and exams done on Friday are less likely to go well than on other days; and that Saturday is the most misjudged and underestimated day.

Rhythm replaces strength.

Sunday: When Does the Week Begin?

Does rest come before or after activity?

Weekend and week beginning

It is clear, isn't it, that the weekend begins on Friday evening and the new week starts again on Monday morning? And yet this division of the week into five working days from Monday to Friday and then two days of weekend leads to problems both of a physical and psychological nature. As the name suggests, we experience the weekend as a well-earned and refreshing end to the week; and the more we enjoy this break, whether by reading, going on excursions or in some other way, the more suddenly and startlingly the new week arrives. This is taxing, and at the same time a good example of the fact that relaxation is often nothing to do with the amount of leisure time we have, but with the organic way in which we structure this time. It is actually part of a healthier way of relating to time that we do not regard Sunday as the last but the first day of the week, as is self-evident in Christian tradition.

Practical consequences

This has practical consequences. If we feel that the new week is beginning on Sunday, we will start looking ahead and thinking about what is coming towards us, and what decisions and plans need to be made. Strengthened by our Sunday rest, we can contemplate the coming week and so allow some of this calm, this inner composure, to flow into the rest of the week.

In his famous statue of David, the sculptor Michelangelo created a work which wonderfully expresses this Sunday mood. Vasari, a biographer of the artist, no doubt sensed something of this when he wrote as follows about the sculpture:

> The diminutive David conquers the giant Goliath with a sling. Why did Michelangelo not express the greatness of this deed by showing in stone how David actually conquers the giant, or even by depicting him

standing in triumph over the fallen giant?

Vasari goes on to say that this is because the greatest moment of David's courageous deed does not lie in the battle itself but in the instant preceding the fight, which Michelangelo sculpts: the moment when David, reflecting, takes his decision; and now all that remains is for his will to stream into his limbs. David's clear, grave and confident gaze expresses more of the soul-mood of Sunday than any number of books.

Hectic stress and calm

Many initiatives, actions and activities would be accomplished in a less hectic, stressful and conflict-ridden way if we could form our resolves on a Sunday. Just as rest is needed after activity so that we relax and reflect, it is also needed beforehand, to collect ourselves for the decisions we are making. The conductor who closes his eyes for a moment before raising his baton; the high-jumper who composes himself before starting his run-up, focusing on his bodily feelings: these are instances of little 'Sunday moments.'

We usually connect rest with relaxation, yet Sunday rest can invoke inner expectancy and excitement about things we are contemplating.

To cultivate Sunday, even perhaps to regard it as sacred, means allowing it to become a sun in our lives. Just as the sun inexhaustibly sends warmth and light to the earth, and thus calls forth life and development, so in Sunday, as the first day of the week, we can find a source of confidence and strength for initiatives that unfold on successive weekdays.

Proverbs such as 'start as you mean to go on' or 'in my end is my beginning' do not suggest that events are predetermined, but rather that, like the seed of a plant, a beginning encapsulates the spirit of an undertaking, endowing it with its intrinsic character. In this sense, Sunday is present throughout the week.

Nowhere, nowhere in the world, is there any lack of participating, approving souls. All that is needed is one whose circumstances leave him entirely free to follow his aims with complete resolve.

Goethe, Clavigo I

Monday: Attending to the New

Can I hold back my response?

Moonrise

The first working day of the week bears the name of the moon for good reason. The moon reveals the quality of devotion in two ways: it is devoted to the sun by reflecting its light and assuming, to our view, the same size as the sun in the heavens; and it is devoted to the earth in that, subduing its own rotation, it couples itself with us and always shows us the same aspect.

In his conversations with Eckermann, Goethe exclaims at one point:

> For heaven's sake, have the courage to attend fully to your impressions, to allow yourself to be delighted, to be instructed also, and to let yourself be kindled and encouraged to accomplish something great ...

In an article on the skills needed in professional biography counselling, I read the following somewhat cutting remark: 'Just sitting there listening is not the same as deep silence.' What the author meant is that far more was needed for openness and empathy in such a therapeutic encounter than a mere invitation to someone to tell their story. It may sound contradictory, but although a therapist has scarcely anything to say in the first few sessions, he must be fully prepared and intimately familiar with the laws of biography. Why? Because at least as much activity can be felt in a person's listening as in their subsequent analysis of another's situation. In seeking to create an open, unprejudiced mood — and this applies to all sorts of other situations — to help the client express himself and find the right words, we have to hold ourselves back. This may sound banal, but it means we must have something specific to hold back. We must have a response to what we hear — our own thoughts, ideas and images — which we are capable of keeping back. The more easily and without obvious effort we manage to hold back our own response, the more richly and trustingly a conversation can develop.

Learning to wonder

In the company of children, particularly, the question continually arises whether we are able to share in their wonder when, for instance, they notice that snails do not pull in their horns in a breeze but do so when you blow on them. Can we keep back our own knowledge in such circumstances?

'Creative spontaneity' makes little sense by itself — it requires some kind of preparation or readiness. This is most noticeable on a Monday. If we experience Sunday as the beginning of the week, using our rest to plan and make decisions about the forthcoming week, Monday can unfold properly. It loses its alarm, and ceases to be the killjoy of the weekend, instead revealing its own intrinsic aspect of bringing something new. On no other day do we encounter so much change as on Monday, and this is why, more than any other day, it requires our openness or even devotion. Yet attending to the new things that Monday brings is only possible when we are looking forward to see whether the ideas we considered on Sunday can be realized on Monday, or whether they were pie in the sky. To find out, we have to absorb reality as far as possible: in other words, allow our own being to grow quiet and at the same time engage it in the greatest activity and attention. This devotion and attention to the outer world is what especially distinguishes the character of Monday.

Openness for Murphy's Law

Naturally, things often go quite differently on Monday than we envisaged the day before; but if we're well enough prepared, our imaginative response will come into play and allow us to cope fruitfully with whatever happens. In this case, Murphy's Law really does apply: if things don't go as planned, be happy that they turned out otherwise.

Attentiveness is in fact not simply a virtue
or the result of upbringing, but a state of
being, without which we could never be
whole. It is, truly, a place where the universe
listens in.

Jaques Lusseyran, The Blind in Society and Blindness: A
New Seeing of the World.

Tuesday: A Special Day for Mistakes

Do we hestiate when
action is called for?

Decisions and plans

Every plan we make, whether to research a country we would like to visit, or a communal project, or landscaping a garden, takes place in phases. These separate, characteristic stages can occur throughout an afternoon or, when time presses, can follow quickly on each other's heels in a matter of minutes. They come to light most clearly however over consecutive days separated by sleep, the most incisive, repeating pause in our lives.

A more or less conscious decision always stands at the outset of a plan or intention. The more far-seeing and carefully pondered this is, the more impetus can flow into the plan, and the less likely doubt and scepticism will be. Once taken, a decision strengthens our inner sense of certainty, diminishing the impact of external problems. This is the Sunday mood: making a new beginning based on calm reflection.

Then comes Monday and resolve encounters actual circumstances. The freer we are from prejudice and the more openly we meet and take account of the reality approaching us, the more organically the new can build on the old. The ideas or ideals of Sunday have to connect with what actually happens. On Monday we can often discover how free or otherwise our relationship with our ideas is: are we in love with them or can we stay true to their kernel and dispense with their superfluous shell? The American business author Bill Emmot describes this modern, change-oriented virtue of letting go and keeping hold simultaneously as 'creative destructiveness.'

Actualized will

Actualized will now grows from the dialogue between decisions and experienced reality. The real work begins. In our example of landscape gardening, the decision, say, to build a curved drystone wall may be blocked by the discovery of a concrete post. On

Tuesday, therefore, we take a pickaxe and set to work to remove the obstruction, forgetting various other factors in the process. Hindrances that we meet are cleared out of the way, and the desire grows on Tuesday to give increasing shape to those Sunday plans. This day is therefore informed by a particular dynamic and approach.

The threefold dynamic of the planet Mars

Among the planets, we associate the character of the third day of the week with Mars. Just as Tuesday is connected with pressing ahead and the urge for action, so the red planet Mars shows the strongest dynamism in the planetary system. It does so in four ways: in the polar opposites of bright-dark, quick-slow, high-low and calm-tempestuous. For long periods it can only be glimpsed as a weakly glinting, orange point of light, but when it approaches more closely to the earth it gleams brighter than Jupiter. Its path is unusually compressed, causing it to alternate between a rapid and slow orbit. Only on Mars do sandstorms sometimes shroud the whole planet. Furthermore, the Olympus Mons on Mars is the highest mountain in the solar system, over three times higher than the Himalayas; and accordingly, at ten kilometres deep, Hellas Planitia is the deepest basin to be found on any of the planets.

The interest of mistakes

Encouraging oneself to pursue and realize one's own ideas also involves creating an atmosphere in which mistakes are not only seen as regrettable but are acknowledged and affirmed as necessary aspects of development. Since unconstrained effort belongs above all to Tuesday, it is particularly important on this day to develop a 'culture of mistakes' and regard errors as interesting.

The person who acts is always without conscience. A conscience is possessed only by those who observe.

Goethe, Maxims and Reflections

Wednesday: Interest in What's Around You

What is a centre
without a periphery?

At work, and after

To make a decision in calmness and composure, with openness for and devotion to actual circumstances in the world, and to realize such decisions with dynamism and commitment, are the typical qualities of Sunday, Monday and Tuesday. What now follows the energy and drive that prevailed on Tuesday?

It is something that can no doubt be observed in all forms of collaboration. Here is an example: we are getting a room ready for a festival, with the help of several others. Each person has taken on a particular task such as laying tables, setting up the buffet or arranging flowers. Before long, usually before our own activity has been accomplished, we start to be interested in what the others are doing or have achieved. Whereas previously each person was occupied in their corner, as though wearing imaginary blinkers, we start going over to look at other people's work. Suddenly several people or maybe all are standing together and looking at something in particular.

Concentration and expanding attention

Here a typical rhythm of the human psyche becomes apparent: from concentrated activity, an interest arises in what is happening around us. What have the others accomplished and how does it correspond with what I myself have done? What in my wider surroundings might be of interest and inspiring for my own work? Such questions are typical motivators on a Wednesday. This is also the reason, for instance, why local meetings of the Anthroposophical Society largely take place on Wednesdays — in an effort to form new insights and initiatives by meeting with other like-minded or spiritually-oriented people. Here we primarily need to pay attention to the work and questions of others. The special potential for this is present on Wednesday, the day of Mercury (as reflected in mercredi, the French for Wednesday).

Mercury the relationship creator

A glance from the quality of Wednesday to the characteristics of Mercury can show that deep wisdom, dating back around 4,000 years, underlies the assignment of planets to the days of the week. No other planet engages in such multi-faceted contact with its surroundings as this nearest planet to the sun. Two of Mercury's distinctive characteristics are that it orbits the sun so fast that it overtakes the earth on average every 116 days. Besides this sun orbit, it also spins on its own axis as all planets do. It takes 58 days to complete one such rotation, exactly half of 116, and thus of the time between one earth encounter and the next. Mercury's rotation is coordinated with the earth; but that is not all. Mercury's average distance from the sun, at 55 million kilometres, is 38% of the earth's distance (149 million kilometres) and its size, measuring 4,880 kilometres in diameter, is likewise 38% of the earth's size (12,740 kilometres). Thus in both size and distance from the sun, Mercury has the same relationship to the earth.

In fact, 38% is the smaller portion of the Golden Section, a ratio which appears in all growth processes and natural forms. Whereas Mercury's orbit and rotation show harmonious musical time relationships such as 1:2 or 2:3, in its distance and size it reflects the creative proportion of the Golden Section (or the divine section as it was called in the Renaissance). However divergent, in fact polar opposite, these temporal and spatial relationships are, they both accord with the fact that the planet has a fruitful, harmonious relationship with its cosmic surroundings.

A further unique quality of this planet underscores the perfection with which Mercury realizes the 'relationship' principle: it places itself freely into its context without tending more in one direction than another. We can take this quite literally: it is the only planet whose axis stands vertically to its orbit without inclining one way or the other. It assumes no prior 'stance' and can therefore enter equally into relationships with all the surrounding planets. Its distinctive quality is to 'enter into relationship with its surroundings' — the mercurial characteristic.

A day for growing

Mercury forms interrelationships with other planets through its spatial orientation and particular type of motion; and attentiveness enables us to do something similar in our own lives. Interest in what's around us, affirming things previously alien, opens up new sources of inspiration. Daily food intake forms the basis for life, for growth. In the same way, external stimulus and the new ideas we gain from it enrich our inner life and encourage spiritual growth.

What is foreign to us has a life that is foreign, and we cannot fully appropriate it if we welcome it immediately and gladly like a familiar guest.

Goethe in a letter to Gottfried Herder

Thursday: Acting with Insight and Overview

How does a correct
judgment become just
and a just verdict wise?

More than just travel nerves

'Have I thought of everything?' When getting ready to go on holiday, this question can assume dire proportions. 'Did I cancel the papers, are the pets taken care of, do I have my passport, is there anything I've forgotten to tell anyone?' Such pre-travel nerves are often a desperate attempt to make sure we haven't forgotten or overlooked anything. Even when we've reassured ourselves, we can easily feel uncertain again a moment later. Some people are so unsettled by this pre-travel restlessness that it spoils any sense of excitement they were feeling about seeing new countries and cultures. Underlying it, often, is the idea that we might forget something that will later come back to haunt us, since it will be too late then to do anything about it. This is true of other situations too, but is accentuated when we're about to go travelling.

In general this feeling is about a failure in the present that will confront us in the future. No doubt one of the most striking examples of this is the misfortune that occurred during manufacture of the Hubble telescope, which was subsequently sent into orbit around the earth. The wrong piece of equipment was used for polishing the primary mirror, giving rise to an erroneous curvature in the mirror's surface. The mistake only became clear once the telescope was already in orbit. A few years ago this error was largely corrected in a laborious and expensive 'telescope rescue mission' during which a corrective mirror was inserted.

Mistaken judgments and their consequences

How does this relate to the human and social realm? The educationalist Rudolf Grosse gives an example from his time working as a teacher. During a teachers' meeting there was a discussion about a difficult pupil, and the teachers pooled their observations about him: he often didn't do his homework, showed little interest in lessons, gazed into the distance, seldom played with his classmates at break-times, and so forth. The teachers concluded together that the pupil was lazy. 'Bone-idle!' added an indignant teacher. Yet soon after, it was not the pupil who stood condemned but the teachers themselves, due to the school doctor's diagnosis: the boy suffered from a severe digestive disorder. His difficulty passing stools affected his capacity to be mentally alert and involved.

This example aims to show that things we overlook in the social domain can be particularly grave since their consequences often cannot be remedied. These mistaken judgments, the moral condemnation of the boy, might easily have a serious impact on his further development. If we examine our own mistaken decisions and actions, we usually find that the mistake does not arise through false observations or ideas but by forgetting to consider something, by failing to take account of an apparently unimportant yet key aspect. We leave something important out of the picture, and this leads to erroneous actions.

Awareness of the broader context: ecology

The fact that we need an awareness of the broader context when making effective decisions in social situations is true particularly of the quality of Thursday. On Wednesdays we can sense the soul's fundamental mood to be enhanced interest in our surroundings, thus creating for Thursday the necessary conditions for actions that take account of wider effects and ramifications. One might in fact call such actions 'ecological,' because ecology is the study of the relationship between organisms and their surroundings. Thursday is therefore particularly suited for acting in a 'socially ecological' way.

In Babylonian times, Thursday was assigned to the planet Jupiter. What distinguishes this giant amongst the planets? Its diameter, at 142,800 kilometres, is almost twelve times that of the earth, and it is twelve times slower in its orbit round the sun. The number twelve always indicates a sense of wholeness and completion. Thus the twelve tribes of Israel, the twelve apostles, the twelve knights of the Round Table or the twelve jurors in a court represent the full range of human diversity — or even the whole of humanity. Correspondingly, we perceive reality through the interplay of twelve separate senses, so our processing of and inner engagement with reality is reflected in twelve possible worldviews. Organization advisors and sociologists therefore often suggest that ideally, to properly evaluate a situation or problem, we should take account of twelve different perspectives.

It is therefore characteristic of this fifth day of the week that we try to develop a full picture in our thinking and act out of this. Put succinctly, the two active, work-accentuating days of Tuesday and Thursday differ in that action and impetus are decisive on the Mars day, whereas on the Jupiter day this is replaced by the possibility of 'wisdom-borne action.'

Men are wise in proportion, not to their experience, but to their capacity for experience.

George Bernard Shaw, A Rebel's Catechism

Friday: The Importance of
What Seems Secondary

How can we make
things beautiful?

Beauty

Our work appears to be finished: we have thought of everything, have considered all circumstances and needs, have even discovered and remedied mistakes. The result is in line with all requirements — and yet one of our colleagues is dissatisfied. He glances over the finished work and makes the surprising suggestion that what has been accomplished still lacks beauty.

It might be a self-built children's play area or a garage for the car. Irrespective of how practical and functional the desired project is meant to be, we wish to add something which is there solely for aesthetic reasons. This represents a desire to liberate ourselves from all necessities and to enhance our work with a special, individual quality drawn from our own creative inspiration. It might be the finishing touch of colour on a wooden shed or a carved shape on the eaves. It might be a pleasing finish to a stone wall in the garden, a vase of flowers on the breakfast table or a special decoration for a cake. Everywhere, in almost every piece of work, a moment arrives when one wishes to place centre stage what is apparently secondary.

Play and imagination

Imagination comes into its own here, allowing us to free ourselves from the diktat of requirements, necessities and conditions. Whereas all practical viewpoints can be derived from prevailing circumstances and originating aims and values — and therefore cannot really be called new — creative enhancement of work gives rise to something new and surprising. It is therefore no wonder that the greatest, childlike enthusiasm is kindled when making something aesthetic. The compliment, 'that's practical' or 'sensible' gives a child much less pleasure, of course, than 'how lovely' or 'that's beautiful.'

Friedrich Schiller's letters on aesthetic education are among the best-known eulogies to imagination: 'For, to say it quite plainly, man only plays where he is, in the full meaning of the word, a human being; and is only fully human where he plays.' In every game we accept self-chosen rules; and in Schiller's view of play, likewise, imagination involves attending to one's own inner feeling of what matches aesthetically, what is harmonious and what not. Without such attentiveness, Schillerian 'play' easily turns to frivolity, and imagination to phantasm. Beauty then only briefly appears original and soon becomes insipid. It may sound paradoxical, but although there are countless ways of beautifying something, arbitrariness is at the same time the enemy of beauty.

The day of beauty and creativity

Friday is the day of the week when we are particularly inclined to elevate our work into an artistic realm. It is preceded by Thursday, when we draw on insight to place things into a broader context. Thursday can render what we do purposeful, while Friday can make it beautiful. Naturally these characterizations should not be followed too rigidly; but they can help us to recognize the different ways in which our work is supported by the week's rhythmic configuration, and times when we are working counter to the qualities of each day. Friday is less suited to trials and tests, because its creative and artistic mood stimulates us to liberate ourselves from external necessities and conditions.

Babylonian cosmology assigns Friday to the planet Venus. In those times, however, it was named Ishtar, the goddess of love and beauty. Subsequent cultures adopted the essence and qualities of this divine being but gave her different names. Ishtar became Aphrodite in Greece, and eventually Venus in Rome. In Teutonic mythology she was called Freya, which gives us the word Friday; in Romance languages the Roman word was retained (French: vendredi).

As Friday is the day of beauty so Venus is the planet of

beauty: no other planet emanates light so generously into its surroundings. Our moon, for example, only reflects 7% of the sunlight it receives, absorbing the rest as warmth. Venus reflects back 70%, which is why it starts gleaming before sunset. If we trace the points in the zodiac through which Venus passes when she is in closer proximity to earth, we produce a regular five-pointed star — a kind of 'cosmic blossom.' This picture recurs on the surface of this bright planet, where meteor strikes have not created typical craters as we know them on the moon and Mercury, but flower-like corona structures. These are caused by lava emerging around craters under the influence of Venus's dense atmosphere.

If Sunday can be called God's day, Friday is that of the creative human being.

Do good, and you nurture the divine
plant of humanity; create beauty and you
scatter seeds of the divine.

Friedrich Schiller, Tabulae Votivae

Saturday: How Does the Old Enter the World?

How well do we
grow old?

Anyone who has attended the performance of a symphony knows the magnificent moment at the end when the last phrase has been played. With a scarcely noticeable movement of both hands the conductor indicates the conclusion of the final note. The music fades and there is an instant of silence — not fractured by impatient applause only because the musicians and the conductor maintain the tension for a second or two with their intense focus. The violinists still hold bows to strings, the wind players keep their mouthpieces at their mouths, and the conductor's gesture seems frozen in time. Then he lowers his arms, relaxes his shoulders and, in a shared exhalation by audience, musicians and conductor, the applause begins. The piece is over. There are probably few other occasions when we can hear such a full, 'pure' silence as that, just after a concert. In these brief seconds the whole symphony seems to be present in concentrated form. The successive melodies, the rise and fall of different phrases suddenly coalesce in this moment of tableau-like simultaneity. Anyone who has experienced music's timelessness in this way will believe Mozart when he writes that some of his symphonies were conceived in an instant, and then required laborious days of work to write down all the parts. Even if this far exceeds normal capacities, it nevertheless characterizes a typical aspect of the human spirit: the ability to bring different and distant phenomena together in a simultaneous whole.

A time for review

The capacity described above can unfold particularly on Saturday when we look back on the past week. Rather than an analytic review, a strict evaluation of what went well and what didn't, this is more like a kind of 'musical remembering.' What does this mean? New relationships and connections between the week's events appear as we juxtapose them with each other, going beyond known causal connections. We can start to trace deeper-lying causes and motives, in which time also seems to be reversed.

For instance, an apparently chance conversation during a train journey on Tuesday may only acquire significance when we find that it bears relation to a task, say, on the following Friday. Thus the reason for the conversation seemed to lie in the future.

On Saturday, the day of Saturn, the week comes to an end. But every period of time, whether a single day or the great cycle of a cultural epoch, shows characteristic phases that start with a new impetus: in a conversation this might be the initial greeting, in the seasonal round it is spring, and for children the new, unwritten school book marking the start of a new school year. In the same way, the end of every developmental cycle is marked by a conclusion: often, by maturation and internalization.

Innovation and maturity

In recent years the question has often been asked: 'How can something new enter the world?' This question addresses the developmental conditions for innovation. What nurtures new ideas; what favours vision and the necessary corrections to the way we are heading? How do we stay fresh; how does a friendship or working group find the energy to renew itself? Only half the answer is contained in what is new, in development's 'starting conditions.' We must equally ask about the old: how can what already exists ripen so that it gives rise to new seeds? How does the old enter the world?

Whereas getting old at the physical level is something that happens by itself, growing old in soul means growing in maturity, which occurs to a much lesser degree by itself. While Sunday stimulates us to make new decisions and form new outlooks, and thus rejuvenates us, Saturday helps us to grow old by striking a chord from the week's diverse events and experiences, and thus 'harvesting' them.

The creative pause

No doubt because our culture today is so fixated on youth, Saturday tends to be the most overlooked day. Leisure activities and the entertainment industry largely occupy the day when it would make most sense to have a creative pause. Though seeking diversion at the weekend is very understandable, it is important to make space for some peace after the ups and downs of the past week. Perhaps we shy away from this peace, too, because it is always somewhat tinged with sadness — sadness that the process, the specific life of this week is now past. Yet little death processes — when the music falls silent for instance, and equally when we look back at the previous week — are illumined by Goethe's saying about great natural cycles: 'Death is life's greatest invention for having still more life.'

On Saturday, as we revive the events of the week in our memory, they can die away in the best sense of the word and transform into personal capacities. Thereby we become free for new experiences and ideas, and are ready for the new Sunday.

And so the circle of the week closes, the sevenfold wingbeat of the soul.

By far the best experience of men is made up of their remembered failures in dealing with others in the affairs of life.

Samuel Smiles, Character

2 | Living with the Rhythms of Time

The Equilibrium of the Present

'Learn to understand what is healthy by looking at what is sick,' stated Rudolf Steiner; and this also applies when we examine our relationship with time. Loss or failure of memory is one of the gravest injuries to our human sense of time or our human existence altogether. Such impairment is widespread of course in milder forms. After concussion, for instance, many people notice that their memory has gaps — that they cannot recall events directly connected with the injury they sustained, as if that time no longer exists and can only, approximately, be experienced through the accounts of others. This little piece of missing past has little impact on our experience of the present, however. It is much more serious when a cerebral haemorrhage deprives someone entirely of the capacity for recall. New impressions or even personal thoughts and feelings can no longer find a purchase in the memory. An impression only lasts in the psyche for the briefest period, scarcely more than twenty seconds, and a veil of forgetfulness shrouds all that is perceived. Such loss of memory means that if you look at the clock, or out of the window to see what the weather's like, or if a friend phones to say he's coming to visit, you forget it all again immediately. You no longer know the origin of the cheerful mood caused by news of a friend's visit, so you assume it is just unfounded cheerfulness. The alarming thing here is that loss of the past also closes off the future: if we can retain nothing in our memory we also lose everything that connects us to the future.

How can this be? Every wish we harbour, every plan we conceive involves an engagement of some kind with the future. We cast a mental fishing line into the future and draw it back into the present. A financial service provider's advert — 'Thinking about the future now' — is well chosen since it applies to far more than merely commercial precautions. The future is always, inevitably, part of our present experience, and every decision, every hope, is directed towards it. In every instant, therefore, seeds germinate towards the future. But in order for them to grow, becoming sources of our actions, we need to protect and preserve them, and this requires memory. It sounds contradictory, but with loss of our memory we can no longer recall our own future.

You might think that this incapacity would liberate us from the freight of memories and visions of the future and allow us to enjoy the present undisturbed, but the opposite is true. Our 'now' is only a rich experience through the presence of past and future. As we digest past experiences and learn to understand new ones, we allow the past to live in the present; and as we set ourselves new aims, we not only think about the future but also create it.

A second apparent contradiction is the following: although it is true that the past and future enrich our present, they can also flood and drown it out. In our experience of the present moment, past and future seem like the two sides of a pair of scales. When they are in balance we feel ourselves 'at home' in the moment. But as soon as one of them preponderates, it becomes hard to really engage in the immediate present. An example from childhood: expectations of Christmas can cause irritation with the intervening period that seems to stand between me and the gifts I'm looking forward to. Worries about the future, or nostalgic memories of a happier past, can overshadow the present. Anyone subject to this feels that the future and past possess a power of their own that can assume excessive proportions in the human soul if we do not continually re-establish a happy medium.

In the zodiac, the sign of the scales stands opposite that of the ram. In almost all illustrations, this ram is depicted in a somewhat unusual stance: it sits facing the circling sun, yet turns its head in the opposite direction. Thus it becomes an image of equilibrium in the temporal realm, a balance between past and future.

By facing the future yet — like the ram — looking back to the past, our present becomes a rich experience.

How Long is the Present?

Many daily gestures such as shaking hands, pointing out a direction, or a welcoming smile, last around three seconds. This corresponds to a single breath, given an average breathing rhythm of twenty breaths per minute. We also clearly sense when we have exceeded this 'moment' because such gestures start to feel forced. Let's look a little closer at this three-second period.

There's a simple test you can try out on yourself, suggested by Ernst Pöppel. Take a metronome (or a dripping water tap) and set it at sixty beats per minute. Each second is marked by one beat. With the least experience of Viennese waltzes, we have no difficulty whatever in hearing this uniform beat as 3/4 time, three beats in a bar — or in other words we inwardly accentuate every third beat. If we take the slowest possible metronome pulse, it is much harder to hear a waltz tune in its monotonous beat, since 3 x 1.5 seconds until the next accented note far exceeds the three-second duration of a breath. Only within this span of time can we easily gain the sense of a bar, a group of beats. Without having to remember, we know when an accent is due again, as all three beats, despite sounding in succession, are 'compiled' in our mind into a present. The same is true in conversation. Even a longer sentence is understood when spoken, without us having to actively recall the beginning of the sentence. The succession of words, and even of syllables, is something we integrate into a non-successive whole. This does become harder, however, if pauses, especially at inappropriate points, exceed the span of three seconds.

'Now' is, in human experience, not just a skin-thin boundary between future and past, between 'in a moment' and 'just now,' but has a temporal duration that only we ourselves produce. The sand-clock as an image of passing time is only therefore appropriate as a physical measure. Soul time does not flow continuously in the same way, but runs in single waves, each of which endures for three seconds as a small parcel of time. The 'now' feeling arises as we merge together successive events into temporal units.

This is why watching and listening to plays, dance or music is a good way to school our sense of time. In these 'time arts,' present moments are created that are longer than the breath. Whether as melodies stretching their arc over many bars, the entirety of a dancer's sequence of movement or an actor's soliloquy, the audience can in response develop more elevated present moments. A drama or a symphony can ultimately transform in the soul to a single, whole presence.

In these higher and more encompassing forms of 'now,' the pervasive diktat of cause and effect, of 'must ... because' is suppressed. The laws of physics and causality pale, and suddenly we can have an artistic experience of a conceivable, opposite realm: a later cause can actually give rise to an earlier event. For instance, two people do not live together because they once got to know each other and came to love one another, but the reverse: they had to meet in order to live together as they do.

Our physically enlightened reason is wrong to prevent us looking at fate as though the cause might lie temporally after the effect. Denying this reality of the reversed stream of time will hinder us from experiencing the magic and wisdom which, despite all chance occurrence and freedom, lives in human destiny.

There are many people who have been revived after a severe accident and who speak of having a near-death experience. Their accounts are unanimous in describing their life passing before them in a tableau, a kind of simultaneous panorama. Neurologists often seek to explain away this phenomenon by saying that all our memories are released at once in the dramatic state of oxygen deprivation. Yet this higher simultaneity is nevertheless supersensible in nature, in the same way as we partake a little of the supersensible realm in the enhanced experience of immediacy we can gain from a symphony, book or play.

> Watching and listening to plays, dance or music is a good way to school our sense of time. In these 'time arts' present moments are created that are longer than the breath.

Speed and Heart Rhythm

For many weeks one summer, the sculptor Mirella Faldey moved into an open wooden shed close to my office and set up her workshop there, creating four open-air sculptures. She had sought out the hardest stone, granite, as her material. To work it you need specially toughened steel chisels which emit a ringing tone when they strike the stone: 'ding, ding, ding.' After four weeks I had got used to this regular, bright sound so that it more or less merged into the other noises in the vicinity. But then came a surprise. One day, suddenly, the chisel strokes disturbed me again, but in a much more penetrating way than on the first day, making me unusually nervous and unfocused. Looking through the window to the shed I saw that a male sculptor had replaced Mirella and was tackling the stone with special energy. Although his chisel strokes were no louder or less regular, I could barely stand the noise. Why? Looking at the clock on the wall gave me the explanation. The assistant sculptor was using his hammer and chisel 170 to 180 times a minute, or in other words three times a second. This was a good deal faster than his colleague, who worked at a calmer tempo of about 140 to 150 strokes a minute. The difference of thirty strokes more per minute seems small, but is decisive. Whereas the slower rhythm still resonates in a somewhat musical fashion, the faster rhythm has an insistent, mechanical quality.

The point at which a rhythm loses its sense of naturalness and ease is due to an elemental human rhythm. Besides the heartbeat rhythm of around 75 beats per minute, there is another heart rhythm, roughly twice as quick, which is caused by the response of blood vessels to the heartbeat, their elastic absorption of the pulse. After every pulse beat the pressure wave spreads from the heart through the arteries into the whole body. The finely branching system of blood vessels reflects the pulse beat back towards the heart and allows the blood to flow back a little. Since the heart chambers are now closed, the blood cannot flow back into them but instead surges from the closed heart back to the periphery of the circulation system. Thus every original heartbeat is followed by the echo of a second, weaker pulse, visible in an ECG as a smaller wave. The blood not only resonates in the pulse rhythm of 75 beats per minute, but also in the double frequency of around 150 beats. This 'overtone' of the blood is known as basic arterial vibration and is the quickest fluctuating rhythm in the body.

But as well as setting a temporal measure in the blood's circulation, basic arterial vibration acts as a temporal sound-reflector in the soul. This is why hardly anyone is likely to wish to, or be able to write a personal letter at the same speed as a phone number noted down in passing. To put our personal stamp on handwriting we need to write no faster than this fundamental resonance allows. Our gait also unfolds within this range. At more than 150 steps per minute, movement becomes mechanical and hectic.

While the heart only beats in the chest in spatial terms, we rediscover its temporal influence in walking, writing, hand-shaking, craft work and music-making — as long as it is not ousted from these activities by excessive speed.

How Long Does a Moment Last?

If we assume a moment to be, literally, the blink of an eye, the answer to this question is six seconds. That's the period of time in which eyelids blink once on average. They slide down rapidly over the eyes, re-distribute the tear fluid, clean the eye's surface and give a brief respite from seeing, a swift moment of rest. Yet this fraction of a second pause in sight is decisive because it rhythmically structures vision. We look out into the world with open eyes, departing from ourselves because our sight takes us out into the phenomena around us, but the eye-blink[1] brings us briefly back to ourselves. It helps us, for instance, to regain a little detachment after complete involvement and absorption, so that we don't entirely lose our capacity for judgment in self-forgetful gazing.

The rhythm of the blinking eye is not only different in each of us but also varies depending on the work we are doing and our inner state of mind. It can speed up to be as quick as the breathing rhythm, with the lids closing every three seconds, or it can slow down to just a few times per minute. The latter is likely in a reverent or contemplative mood, whereas in a heated discussion or when we feel uncertain, the eyes can blink frantically.

We can do a little test on ourselves: if we look at nature or at a painting and blink frequently as we do so, we find that a certain

---

[1] In German the word Augenblick (literally 'eye-blink') means 'moment.'

span of uninterrupted vision is needed for us to work through an impression in our feelings. Too frequent blinking prevents us fully absorbing or participating in something new.

The eyes are always involved in absorbing information, are intellectually challenged, whether we're driving, working at a computer or reading. It is advisable to balance this by allowing the eyes to dream, too, from time to time — in other words to let colours and forms pervade them. The eyes have to grow calm in order to enjoy the yellow of a blossoming rape field or the colour nuances of a sunset. This seems to happen by itself the moment we turn to such an impression in a focused but open way.

The psyche configures the body's temporal sequences to suit its activity. As the physician and cosmologist Walter Bühler puts it, the body becomes the instrument of the soul. The blinking eye is a kind of soul breathing. It grows calmer in a reverent mood, and its frequency increases with intellectual activity, for instance when we're trying to find our way in an unknown area, or when we're looking for something we've lost.

In Bertolt Brecht's play *Galileo*, the dramatist has the Italian astronomer explain to his housekeeper how the movements of the planets should be seen heliocentrically. To demonstrate this he sits her on a swivel chair and starts spinning it. When he asks her what she saw she gazes at him with incomprehension, and he flares up at her, saying, 'You shouldn't just stare, you should look!' He means that we can only understand what we see by briefly turning away after observing something: then the immediate impression recedes and space is created for thinking.

After blinking we look out again afresh into the world. The six-second blinking rhythm amounts to 5,000 moments of fresh vision every day. The blink of an eye is therefore sleep's little brother, just as sleep itself is known as the little brother of death. As we blink, the ongoing process of sight 'dies,' but that is precisely what makes it human. Just as we rediscover ourselves anew after a night's rest, and can then look on the world again with new eyes, so every blink renews our eyesight.

One of the most charming ways of greeting someone is with a wink, as the renewal and refreshing of sight is not for our own sake but for another.

After blinking we look out again afresh into the world.

The New Day Begins
in the Evening

Transitions that involve passing from one state to another, from one form of life to a different one, are the most spiritually active moments. We often only notice this later, since only in the safe haven of the new phase of life does it become clear how lively and active the period of change was. What may have been experienced at the time as uncertainty or crisis is later revealed as a phase of special intensity.

Such transitions may be major stages of development, such as that from youth to adulthood, from training to the practice of a profession and family life, or in advancing towards old age when various personal and societal responsibilities are gradually taken from our shoulders. But besides these periods of major change, our biographical path seems to hold its breath and intensify at other moments. On a smaller scale, too, human time is configured in differentiated ways, and made rhythmic by intervals and pauses. This happens most regularly in the alternation between day and night, between waking and sleeping. Comparable to the bar lines of a piece of music, this rhythm forms a fundamental oscillation in human life. Here too, the transition moments between these polar states have a particularly intense quality.

In the same way that sunrise and sunset offer the greatest wealth of colours in the day, this transitional, gloaming period offers us special possibilities. Nature cools and comes to rest at twilight, and the same is true of us. Our pulse and breathing grow slower from late afternoon onwards, blood pressure sinks, and our speed of reaction slows. A decisive change also occurs in the body's warmth system: while temperature sinks at the forehead and internally, it rises in the hands and feet. Just as the earth rays out the heat of the day into the cosmos, our own body heat likewise turns towards the periphery. We therefore need to keep ourselves warmer than in the morning.

But as well as our need of warmth and sensitivity to cold, our awareness of noise also rises in the evening. As light fades, not only our warmth expands but also our hearing capacity. Sounds from afar now reach the ears. Every creak in the house or noise from the street is perceived more attentively. These phenomena accentuate our experience that in the evening the soul releases itself from close focus, from the day's preoccupations, to widen and expand. This is why we are especially receptive to 'food for the soul and spirit' during evening hours. This might involve a concert or trip to the theatre, inviting guests for a meal, a short walk or reading an interesting book. The evening is the time when we are most able to discover new questions or absorb different perspectives.

In the evening, the day's events can once more be invoked. While an exciting crime-thriller film may 'rivet' us, cultural events in the evening, a concert or theatrical performance, can support this expansion of the soul and can often act as catalysts to help us draw some reflective profit from the day's events. However paradoxical it sounds, this occurs primarily through questions. The best harvest of the day is if something we experienced appears to us as a riddle in the evening and loses a little of its apparently self-evident quality; for questions about the way things are always mark the start of new development. This applies not only to doubt and scepticism, which question things in a disengaged or dismissive way, but more to questions with some aim, some personal connection — which always, whether we know it or not, inherently contain something of their answer.

From Discoverer to Philosopher in the Cycle of the Year

In the seventies, the German railways launched investigations into the frequency of errors made by engine drivers. Were there particular times when signals were more often overlooked and top speeds exceeded? The company found the well-known phenomenon that most mistakes occur in the early afternoon, between two and three p.m. At this time of day there is the greatest risk of briefly falling asleep. A full stomach after lunch is not the prime reason for this, since people showed symptoms of exhaustion even if they ate no lunch. The railway investigators also discovered that, following the introduction of a day off on Saturday, trains were more often delayed on Mondays. After two work-free days, the organism has to adjust again to work, and this, according to rhythm researcher Gunther Hildebrand, was what led to the operational problems.

But besides these two times of increased tendency for errors and exhaustion — the 'low-point' in the afternoon, and on Mondays — the investigators found a fluctuating performance graph through the year: in December, January and February a third more errors occurred compared to the same length of time in spring (April/May) and the start of the autumn (October), when there were least.

Central heating, imported vegetables and fruit from southern lands in the winter, and air-conditioning in the summer, detach us from our connection with the seasons. The enquiries of rhythm research can help us to take proper account of the seasonal cycle as a series of temporal transitions reflected not only in the leaves on the trees and the length of the days but also in our mental and physical state. A few examples can illustrate this. During the winter months our reaction times are slowest. We respond relatively dully to external stimulus and there is also a widespread tendency to resignation and despondency. What do the findings of rhythm research tell us here? They show not only that physical performance is greater in summer but also our capacity to gain physical and mental stimulus and inspiration from the external world. In the winter, the external world's influence grows weaker. Our sensory activity fades in autumn as nature comes to rest and the life forces in perennial plants and trees withdraw. With the dark time of year, our attention turns from our surroundings back to ourselves. Whereas we immerse our souls in summer in nature's diversity, in growth, blossoming and the humming of bees, and in our fellow human beings with whom we converse, in winter we withdraw more, instead, into the cosmos of our own souls. In summer we tend more to be discoverers, in winter philosophers and artists. The fact that rhythm research comes up with mostly negative findings for the winter, as stated above, is due to the difficulty in measuring this seasonally-governed philosophizing and artistic sensibility. That reaction times are slower in winter should not lead us to conclude that we are sleepier. In fact the opposite is the case: in winter we are wide awake because we are fully in ourselves.

In winter's peace and interiority we develop our steadfastness. By drawing on the potential of this season for self-reflection, and pondering on our relationship with worlds above us, we create the foundation for fully engaging again in the dynamic activity of spring and summer.

On the arena of the human soul, therefore, summer and winter join hands. In nature, the seeds of autumn and winter start pushing into growth in spring, forming relationships with their surroundings through roots and leaves. In the same way we lay soul-spiritual seeds in winter, which can become reality in spring and summer.

Ex-Beatle George Harrison, who died in November 2001, coined the following phrase: 'Everything else can wait but the search for God cannot.' We can give this phrase special importance in the dark months of winter.

Everything else can wait but the search for God cannot.

The Will's Small and
Great Rhythm

'The greater is reflected in the smaller' is a prime law of living things. For instance, as well as seeing human soul activity in relation to the human body — so that the head equates with thinking, the chest with feeling and the limbs with will — we can go further and seek all three realms of the psyche in the head itself. Then we find that the forehead corresponds to thinking; nose, eyes and mouth, as the centre of the head, express feeling; and the chin and jaw as the head's only moveable part correspond to will. The hand is another example. We grasp, point and hold things with it, and so it is an instrument of the will; and yet the fingertips possess a perceptive capacity typical of our head and thinking. The expressive quality of the palm and back of the hand in gestures shows that this region is dominated by feeling. That's why we find it strange if, when shaking hands with someone, they only take hold of the front part of our hand, the fingers. In greeting someone the hand surfaces have to meet so that we briefly perceive each other there. The thumb is really the only inherently will-oriented part of the hand.

The whole is reflected in the part: this is a characteristic of every living thing, not just in relation to its spatial but also its temporal form. Thus in nature, the great structures of time can be found in small ones. Differing measures of time are related to each other in the same way as the course of the year and the day. What we experience as freshness and cheerfulness in the morning corresponds to spring in the seasons' round. Spring is the year's morning, and therefore the Easter festival has a morning quality while Christmas is a night-time festival. In the same way we can sense a connection between summer and midday, and the afternoon and autumn.

But there is a less familiar relationship between two human rhythms: the moon takes exactly one hour to move the distance of its own diameter across the backdrop of the stars. The same time is needed for something strange or new to become fully a part of us. Whatever we preoccupy ourselves with for an hour, whether a thought, an artwork or a plant can, to the extent we manage this, take such deep root that it makes us into a different person. This is the rhythm of the human will. If we take an hour to think about someone else, our relationship with him can acquire lasting depth and honesty.

We can ask whether this will rhythm of an hour (or 1/24 of a day) corresponds to a comparable period at the level of a whole human life. The calculation produces this result: 72 years divided by 24 = 3. What the hour represents in the day corresponds therefore to three years in a life. If we think of the first three years of life, of early childhood development, we see that everything which we need later in life is formed then: walking, speaking, thinking, use of the senses and, as the crowning quality, the ability to experience oneself as an individual, as 'I.' This breathtakingly quick development occurs — and this is the mysterious thing — without parents having much influence on when and how each step takes place. Neither the will of the child nor the will of the parents makes the child tirelessly practise grasping, crawling or standing. This is cosmic will at work, a gift of the heavens, a festival that lasts three years. It mirrors the archetypal span of time from the Jordan baptism to Good Friday three years later.

The Quiet Heart

Putting Stress In Its Place

Peter Gruenewald

This book describes a highly effective approach to stress management and personal development. Using heart-based exercises that help manage and transform extreme emotions, it is possible to deal with many forms of stress, anxiety and depression, without resorting to drugs or psychotherapy.

This updated version contains new relaxation and self-motivation exercises, and a wider variety of case studies demonstrating real results. This book is an essential read for anyone who wants to take their physical and emotional health into their own hands.

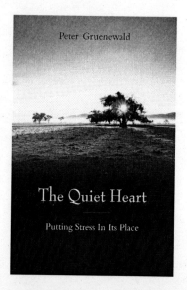

florisbooks.co.uk